It's Time To Take Off Weight, Feel Great & Keep It Off!
A Journey to Your Best Self

It's Time To Take Off Weight, Feel Great & Keep It Off!
A Journey to Your Best Self

By Randi Light

Published by Enlightened Living, Inc.
Copyright © 2015

Copyright © 2015 by Randi Light

All rights reserved. This book or any portion thereof may not be reproduced or used in any manner whatsoever without the express written permission of the publisher except for the use of brief quotations in a book review or scholarly journal.

ISBN 978-1-944243-30-2

Published by

Enlightened Living Hypnosis, Inc.
37 Shore Drive
Ogden Dunes, IN 46368

www.EnlightenedLivingInc.com

Ordering Information:

Special discounts are available on quantity purchases by corporations, associations, educators, and others. For details, contact the publisher at the above listed address.

U.S. trade bookstores and wholesalers: Please contact Enlightened Living Hypnosis, Inc. at (219) 929-8726 or email randilight@gmail.com.

BRING THIS GUIDE BOOK TO YOUR SESSIONS

Hello Friend,

Welcome Aboard! I honor you for taking this transformational journey. Research clearly demonstrates that self-care helps us to heal and moves humanity forward at the same time. My intentions for this guidebook are to make it easy for you to keep track of your coaching, learning and hypnotic experiences.

Your mind is powerful, creative and virtually untapped. Our work together will give you opportunities to see things in ways you have never seen. This work provides a framework for 'aha' moments, intuitive insights, emotional clearing and deep healing. Our work together could possibly be one of your most life changing experiences. This is the time to heal emotionally, physically, mentally, financially, physically, sexually and spiritually.

Your Journey includes the _Essential 4,_ a proprietary system designed to help you easily and confidently create your goals, achieve your goals and heal in every way:

- The Stress Relief & Confidence Building Session – This session is designed to reduce stress, create more confidence and helps you respond resourcefully to life's challenges. It teaches you how to utilize your mind and begins the journey of emotional clearing in a light, easy and creative way.

- The Regression to the Root Cause Session – The cornerstone of success as it provides an opportunity for deep healing and transformation to take place on the cellular level. You heal your history and reframe your experiences, which allows you to create a bright and compelling future.

- Time Line Therapy with Regression to Limiting Belief Session – This session guides you to releasing a dominant limiting belief that may be blocking you from having the life, money, health and relationships you truly deserve. This allows you to show up in your life as your best self.

- The Forgiveness Fire ™ Session – Forgiveness is key because it frees you. It helps you let go of the pain, resentment and guilt so healing can take place. In essence, all the confidence building and emotional clearing is preparing you for the ultimate healing opportunity – forgiveness, acceptance and letting go.

To Your Success and Happiness, ☺

Randi Light

Randi Light

Set Your Intentions

Decide right now what you want to get from our work together – When you want to hit a target you must know what that target is and then begin to see it clearly! Writing or stating your intentions out loud or to yourself can and usually does change the outcome of an event. The thing is you are setting your intentions either consciously or subconsciously. So take the bull by the horns and decide what you want to have, be or feel from our work together. Always write or state your intentions in the positive.

1 _____

2 _____

3 _____

Remember you can SET YOUR INTENTIONS every day: before a phone call, a meeting, a date, a party, a game, talking to your partner, child or boss, and so much more.

Reasons why it's important that I commit to reading this guidebook, and reflecting on my experiences with hypnosis and use the tools I learn:

1 _____

2 _____

3 _____

4 _____

5 _____

NOTES

Design Your Authentic Self!

Do you know what you want, what you really really want? Sometimes we know what we want and other times we don't. The first step in getting from where you are to where you want to be is getting clear on what you want and why you want it. This exercise is designed to help you get out of your head, and get your body and mind aligned in a fun and creative way.

Who are you one year after working together to achieve your goals?

In just a moment, close your eyes and picture yourself walking along a beautiful and relaxing beach. Imagine, you are enjoying the warmth of the sun, the gentle breeze and the sweet sound of the water flowing in and out. Next, imagine someone in the distance walking towards you. Notice how much you admire this person. All of the sudden you realize it's you, your future self, coming towards you. You appreciate the inner and outer beauty radiating from your future self. You appreciate everything, the clothes, the body and the confidence. You feel connected to this future self and feel extremely grateful you achieved your goals.

Describe who you meet on _____
(write today's date here)

Describe in detail, who you meet that day; the size you are, the clothes you wear, the thoughts you think, the feelings you experience. What you do and what you don't do. Include all the things you have accomplished and created emotionally, physically, mentally and spiritually.

___
___
___
___
___
___
___
___
___
___
___
___
___
___
___
___
___
___
___
___
___

How you are going to become this you!

STEP 1 - Commit! Make a clear decision right now. Answer these 2 questions.

Are you ready to change? _____

Are you willing to change? _____

I agree from this moment forward to be on the path to a healthier and happier me!_____
Sign your name

WRITE DOWN EVERYTHING YOU EAT AND DRINK FOR 3 DAYS. BE SPECIFIC. START RIGHT NOW!

Day 1	Day 2	Day 3

Mindset. Food. Fitness.

STEP 2

As a result of the work you are doing you will naturally feel more in control of your thoughts, feelings, actions and habits. If you fall into an old behavioral pattern, recognize it (don't judge it), learn from it and take charge. Below is a list of ideas you can choose to put into action to Take Off Weight, Feel Great and Keep It Off!

As you read through the different ideas, put a check mark ☑ next to the ones that appeal to you. Eventually you will get more specific but for now just pick ones that you would consider doing.

MINDSET ACTION STEPS

- ☐ Visualize yourself the way you want to look and feel for at least one minute every day.
- ☐ Commit to learning to love and accept yourself just the way you are.
- ☐ Listen to a weight loss MP3/CD as close to daily as possible.
- ☐ Get an accountability partner and call each other a minimum of once or twice a week.
- ☐ Get clear on your 'Eating' and 'No Eating Zones.'
- ☐ Stay calm and confident. Nurture yourself. Believe in you!
- ☐ Stay off the scale. Measure your body.
- ☐ Let urges flow in and out just like thoughts. Remind yourself if you really want it you can have it later or tomorrow.
- ☐ You are in control, take charge of that old sabotaging part of you and just say NO! I've got this.
- ☐ Do the Daily Gratitude Exercise.
- ☐ Practice the Self-Hypnosis process to get relaxed and so you can visualize and materialize your goals!
- ☐ Create a success affirmation/declaration that you repeat 20 times in a row 2 x per day.
    - Examples: *I feel full & satisfied on less food. I eat less and enjoy it more. I am calm, confident and in control. My body is getting thinner and healthier. I love moving my body. It feels great to be moving my body again.*

Add your own ideas here

- ☐ _____
- ☐ _____
- ☐ _____
- ☐ _____

Re-write all the mindset action steps that you checked or wrote in the lines.

FOOD ACTION STEPS

- ☐ Chew each bite of food 10 times.
- ☐ Use a smaller plate, especially at dinner.
- ☐ Avoid eating after 7:00 pm.
- ☐ Listen to a weight loss MP3/CD as close to daily as possible.
- ☐ Before eating ask yourself this, 'Am I actually hungry or just bored?'
- ☐ Next time you want to eat 'cake' or drink alcohol, ask yourself this!
  - "Do I really want these 'potato chips' or do I really want to be a size '8?'
  - "Do I want to be a 'couch potato' or do I really want to be a size (___)?"
- ☐ When you go to a restaurant, immediately put ½ of your food in a "to go" box.
- ☐ Stay off the scale the first month - its inches that count.
- ☐ Just Say NO! Or take a small bite or slice of things you believe will sabotage your goals.
- ☐ Avoid carbonated beverages especially diet drinks. Aspartame makes you crave sugar and hold onto fat.
- ☐ Eat a protein and vegetable filled breakfast.
- ☐ Eat whole foods.
- ☐ Eat a small amount of protein with each meal.
- ☐ Purchase a Weight Loss System like Jenny Craig or Seattle Sutton or go to Weight Watchers.
- ☐ Do a 21 day cleanse of no dairy, gluten, soy, and processed sugar.
- ☐ Drink Water - Before you do anything and especially before you eat or drink anything! Squeeze in a lemon or lime to add variety and to alkalize your body.
- ☐ Drink a minimum of half your body weight in ounces of water every day.
- ☐ Eat a healthy snack/small meal every 2-4 hours to keep you blood sugar stable and metabolism functioning optimally.
- ☐ Eat more fruit snacks
- ☐ Eat more vegetable snacks

<u>Add other ideas here</u>

- ☐ _____
- ☐ _____
- ☐ _____
- ☐ _____
- ☐ _____

RE-WRITE ALL THE FOOD ACTION STEPS THAT YOU CHECKED OR WROTE IN THE LINES.

FITNESS ACTION STEPS

- ☐ Walk almost every day for 30 minutes and increase it weekly.
- ☐ Park farther away.
- ☐ Listen to a weight loss MP3/CD as close to daily as possible.
- ☐ Almost always take the Stairs.
- ☐ Hire a Personal Trainer.
- ☐ Join with a running group.
- ☐ Go to the gym.
- ☐ Work out at home.
- ☐ Get an exercise buddy to workout, walk or run together.
- ☐ Take a 'fitness' class (Zumba, Yoga, etc)
- ☐ Use your exercise equipment – Create a plan.
- ☐ Do 20 pushups and 20 sit-ups every other day.
- ☐ Get an accountability buddy and call each other a minimum of once a week.

<u>Add other ideas here</u>

- ☐ _____
- ☐ _____
- ☐ _____
- ☐ _____
- ☐ _____

RE-WRITE ALL THE FITNESS ACTION STEPS THAT YOU CHECKED OR WROTE IN THE LINES.

STEP 3

CHOOSE THE 6 MOST IMPORTANT ACTION STEPS FROM ALL 3 CATEGORIES THAT YOU COMMIT TO DO FOR TWO WEEKS. WRITE THEM AS AFFIRMATIONS.

Example: "I always picture myself at my new goal weight of 220."

1. _____

2. _____

3. _____

4. _____

5. _____

6. _____

Start with these 6 action steps. The goal is to concentrate on doing these 6 for two weeks. Once you've developed these action steps into daily habits, start on another 6 action steps.

Notice there is a daily tracker for you to record your successes. Write your action steps and check (or mark with a smiley face) the daily boxes.

Also, in the Appendix, you will find more of the Action Step Tracker sheets for you to copy and use.

Enjoy!

ACTION STEP #1 (WRITE AS AN AFFIRMATION)

_____
_____

TODAY'S DATE _____

Use the form below to track the days you complete your action step listed above. *Track your progress with check marks, smiley faces or any other way that makes you feel proud of yourself!*

SUN	MON	TUES	WED	THURS	FRI	SAT

===

ACTION STEP #2 (WRITE AS AN AFFIRMATION)

_____
_____

TODAY'S DATE _____

Use the form below to track the days you complete your action step listed above. *Track your progress with check marks, smiley faces or any other way that makes you feel proud of yourself!*

SUN	MON	TUES	WED	THURS	FRI	SAT

===

ACTION STEP #3 (WRITE AS AN AFFIRMATION)

_____
_____

TODAY'S DATE _____

Use the form below to track the days you complete your action step listed above. *Track your progress with check marks, smiley faces or any other way that makes you feel proud of yourself!*

SUN	MON	TUES	WED	THURS	FRI	SAT

ACTION STEP #4 (WRITE AS AN AFFIRMATION)

_____
_____

TODAY'S DATE _____

Use the form below to track the days you complete your action step listed above. *Track your progress with check marks, smiley faces or any other way that makes you feel proud of yourself!*

SUN	MON	TUES	WED	THURS	FRI	SAT

ACTION STEP #5 (WRITE AS AN AFFIRMATION)

_____
_____

TODAY'S DATE _____

Use the form below to track the days you complete your action step listed above. *Track your progress with check marks, smiley faces or any other way that makes you feel proud of yourself!*

SUN	MON	TUES	WED	THURS	FRI	SAT

ACTION STEP #6 (WRITE AS AN AFFIRMATION)

_____
_____

TODAY'S DATE _____

Use the form below to track the days you complete your action step listed above. *Track your progress with check marks, smiley faces or any other way that makes you feel proud of yourself!*

SUN	MON	TUES	WED	THURS	FRI	SAT

THINGS I USED TO DO THAT I RARELY DO, THINK EAT OR DRINK
Examples: Be mean to myself. Sit on the couch for more than 1 hour. Have continuous negative thoughts. Eat bacon. Drink soda. Eat in my car.

I'M IN CHARGE. I'VE GOT THIS. I AM DONE WITH:

___
___
___
___
___
___
___
___
___
___
___
___
___
___
___
___

The Essential 4

Change the Focus of Your Thoughts

DESCRIBE YOUR BEST QUALITIES — YOUR GIFTS · THE AUTHENTIC YOU!

Encouraging, optimistic, patient, kind, generous, helpful, sweet, funny, cool, amazing, intelligent, smart, special, unique, powerful, courageous, spiritual, influential, calm, confident, wonderful, delightful, outstanding, hardworking, enthusiastic, capable, determined, strong, compassion, passionate, loving, giving, caring, amazing, spiritual, joyful.

I am _____	I am _____
I am _____	I am _____
I am _____	I am _____
I am _____	I am _____
I am _____	I am _____
I am _____	I am _____
I am _____	I am _____
I am _____	I am _____
I am _____	I am _____

Loving, accepting, and believing in yourself is fundamental to your success. Focus only on your strengths and your positive qualities. This will bring more confidence and authenticity into your life.

DESCRIBE MEMORIES THAT GIVE YOU A CONFIDENT, SUCCESSFUL OR HAPPY FEELING

You may have been confident in an art project, a test you took, the way you handled a situation, an athletic performance or....?

_____
_____
_____
_____
_____
_____
_____
_____
_____
_____

The Empowering Bracelet Process

1. Put your bracelet on your wrist.

2. When you catch yourself saying something negative about yourself (or the world), say, 'STOP,' picture a big red stop sign in your mind.

3. IMMEDIATELY say something positive and truthful.
   (There are schools of thought that believe we have 17 seconds to change out negative thought to something positive.)

4. Take your bracelet off of your wrist and put it on the other wrist.

Repeat this process with the goal of keeping the bracelet on the same wrist for 1 day and then eventually one week.

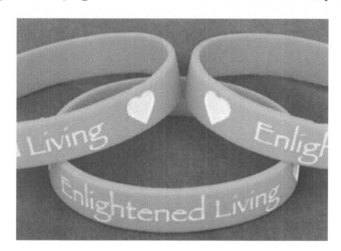

WRITE AND DESCRIBE IN DETAIL 2 DIFFERENT MEMORIES WHEN YOU FELT CALM, CONFIDENT, STRONG, SUCCESSFUL OR HAPPY.

All of us have had moments of 'success,' moments where we felt really proud, strong, wise, or confident. We can access that great feeling by remembering the experience. You may have felt confident because you helped someone or because of how you handled yourself in a situation. For you, maybe you passed a test or created something you liked. It's time for you to remember some of these moments and write them down so you can 'relive' them and feel that great feeling over and over.

_____
_____
_____
_____
_____
_____
_____
_____
_____
_____

Step into Your Power - Stop the Negativity

FOLLOW THE INSTRUCTIONS BELOW TO PROGRAM NEW EMPOWERING THOUGHTS INTO YOUR SUBCONSCIOUS MIND.

Step 1. Write down some of the negative thoughts you find yourself repeatedly thinking in your mind.
Step 2. Then go back and change the thought to something more in line with an outcome or result you want.

Write what pops into your head that is negative. Also throughout your day, pay attention to your thoughts and when you catch yourself saying something negative to yourself or out loud, make a mental note or find your guidebook and write it down.

Here are some examples: (Please note that the positive statement can be a different topic than the negative.)

Negative thought pattern	Positive or grateful thought pattern
I hate when my spouse says that.	I am grateful that my spouse helps me bring in the groceries.
I hate paying my bills.	I am so glad I have the money to pay my bills.
My boss sucks.	My boss is doing the best she can with what she knows.
My child is	I am so grateful my family is healthy
Why am I always in pain?	What can I do to help my body feel better?

Negative Thought_____

Positive Thought_____

Negative Thought_____

Positive Thought_____

Negative Thought_____

Positive Thought_____

Negative Thought_____

Positive Thought_____

Negative Thought_____

Positive Thought_____

Negative Thought_____

Positive Thought_____

Negative Thought_____

Positive Thought_____

The 4 L's: Learn. Laugh. Let It Go. Love Yourself!

How to Get Out of A Negative State Quickly

LEARN–When you look at the world from the perspective that there are no mistakes only learning experiences or that there is no failure only feedback, you free yourself up to learn from the experience. When you can take a positive learning from the situation you can move on and let it go.

When you are dealing with a person or situation that upsets you, ask yourself, <u>"What can I learn from this?"</u>

Write what you could now learn from 2 past experiences that bothered you in some way.

_____
_____
_____

LAUGH – Laughing releases chemical endorphins that can instantly make you feel good. When you can see the humor in the drama of life, and laugh at your own behaviors, and other peoples too, it changes your state to a more resourceful one. Let's face it; sometimes life throws us a lot to deal with at the same time. We are human, we make mistakes, slip-up and say things we wish we could instantly take back. You have a choice in how you respond so...

Ask yourself, <u>"Can I see any humor that I couldn't see before?"</u>

Write down any humor you can now see in your own behavior or someone else's.

_____
_____
_____

LET IT GO– When you learn or laugh at an event, person or situation, you can move on and change how you feel very fast. You automatically change the focus of your thoughts and can let 'it' go. You could literally 'pull' the negative feeling out of your body or you can imagine a big heavy backpack sliding off your shoulders and down your back. Now take an empowering step forward lighter and freer.

LOVE YOURSELF – Start where you need to start, either you love and accept yourself or you learn to love and accept yourself just the way you are. Loving yourself begins with making a commitment to stop criticizing yourself and agreeing to focus on your positive qualities. Become your own BFF (Best Friend Forever).

I promise to stop criticizing myself._____
Sign your name

Do you need ideas to help you love yourself even more?

- *Hearth Breathe*
    1. *Imagine breathing in and out through your heart.*
    2. *Invite your heart to open and see it open, like a rosebud opening into a beautiful green rose or imagine a door opening, tunnel flowing or vortex spinning.*
    3. *Relive a memory when you felt very loving or loved. Relive the loving memory over and over. Feel the loving (or grateful) feeling and breathe it into your heart and into every cell.*

- *Look into a mirror every day for one week and state the following statement out loud, 5 or more times.*

    "I love and accept you _____ just the way you are. (**Write your name on the line.**)

Observe Instead of Judge

What you are habitually thinking about, focusing on and dwelling upon has a tremendous impact on your life because it controlling how you feel, how you act and the types of experiences that show up in your life.

BECOME AWARE OF WHAT YOU THINK ABOUT THROUGHOUT YOUR DAY.

It is estimated that we think up to 60,000 thoughts a day! If just one quarter of your thoughts are negative and unconstructive that's 15,000 thoughts a day focusing on what you don't like, don't want and what you can't do.

Negative thinking can easily activate the fight or flight response in our bodies causing large doses of adrenaline and cortisol to be released. The 'Fight, Flight or Freeze' response is designed to protect you from danger. If a bear is chasing you, your body's fight or flight response is highly effective but when you are mean to yourself or are worried about your in-laws coming over, these chemicals can wreak havoc in your body, mind and life.

When you are continually worried, fearful or overwhelmed your body manufactures the hormones adrenaline and cortisol. Your body cannot simultaneously manufacture the feel good chemicals like serotonin and dopamine at the same time it is manufacturing cortisol, therefore, even small things can make you feel more worried, afraid or frustrated. This learned pattern of thinking leads you to spend your day feeling negative instead of positive, afraid instead of calm, worried instead of peaceful. Anything that is learned can be relearned, unlearned and changed.

You can begin to create new positive patterns of thinking by paying close attention to your thoughts.

Become the OBSERVER INSTEAD OF THE JUDGE. Notice if your thoughts are focusing on what you want or what you don't want; what you like or what you don't like; what you can do or what you can't do.

CHANGE YOUR FOCUS – TRAIN YOURSELF TO THINK ABOUT AND DWELL UPON:

WHAT YOU WANT ~ WHAT YOU LIKE ~ WHAT YOU CAN DO ~ WHAT YOU ARE GRATEFUL FOR

♥ **WHAT I WANT**

_____
_____
_____

♥ **WHAT I LIKE**

_____
_____
_____

♥ **WHAT I CAN DO**

_____
_____
_____

♥ **WHAT I AM GRATEFUL FOR**

_____
_____
_____

DATE _____ **HYPNOSIS SESSION #** _____

My Experiences and insights from the hypnosis:

_____
_____
_____
_____
_____
_____
_____
_____
_____
_____
_____
_____
_____
_____
_____
_____
_____
_____
_____
_____
_____
_____
_____

<u>After the hypnosis session I felt:</u>

_____
_____
_____

Affirming Statements or Mottos I will now verbalize every day:

_____
_____

I promise myself I will:

* _____
* _____
* _____

Conscious Mind vs. Subconscious Mind

In simplified terms, we have two minds, conscious and subconscious. Your conscious mind is reading this and analyzing this information. You can accept the information by thinking, 'Oh yes that makes sense.' Or reject it by thinking, 'No way, that's ridiculous.'

Your conscious mind delivers suggestions to your subconscious mind through habitual thinking. If you habitually assume something is true, even though it may be false, your subconscious will begin to accept it as true.

Most people habitually think negative thoughts instead of positive, uplifting ones. Negative thoughts produce negative feelings and images, whichcan kick in the fight/flight response in the body. When you state out loud or in your mind, "I'm tired" or "I'm overwhelmed" you are delivering a suggestion to your subconscious mind. Repetitive thoughts condition or program your mind for what you want or don't want.

You draw conclusions about your life events that may or may not be true. You give meaning to everything. In essence you create a belief about every life experience; beliefs about yourself, the organization, your family, the world, men, women, etc.

Conscious Mind

- You think approximately 60,000 thoughts a day, every day.
- Your conscious mind looks, listens, learns, analyzes and makes decisions.
- Your conscious mind can accept or reject words, people and opinions.

Subconscious Mind

- Scientific Research has discovered that 95% of our behaviors are subconscious.
- Your Subconscious Mind runs all your bodily functions.
- It can process 4 billion bits of information in 1 second, every second.
- Every memory, even when you were in your mother's womb, is stored in your subconscious, in your nervous system.
- Your subconscious mind stores memories and beliefs from the perspective of the age that you are when the event takes place.

A 4 year-old's version of the world is completely different than a 10 year old, 20 year old or 40 year old. If your parents take your siblings or cousins somewhere and you don't get to go, the 4 year-old you draws a conclusion. The little you may decide 'I am not loved' or 'there must be something wrong with me.' Little you creates a belief, from the viewpoint of the 4 year old self - whether it's true or not.

Conscious Mind	Subconscious Mind
+Linear – one thing after another	+Not limited, deals with everything simultaneously
+Logical	+Intuitive
+Asks, "Why?"	+Knows why
+Intellectual, analytical, cognitive thinking	+Is free to do all the "Feeling"
+Deliberate	+Automatic
+Tries to understand your problems	+Knows the solutions
+Verbal and limited	+Nonverbal, imaginative, expansive
+Focuses on 7 +/- 2 chunks of information at any given time.	+Is aware of everything else
+Processes 2,000 bits of information per second	+Processes about 100 billion bits of info/sec
+These impulses travel about 100-150 mph	+These impulses travel up to 100,000 mph

How our subconscious mind gets programmed

1) What we repeatedly say over and over in our mind.

2) What others repeatedly say to us over and over.

3) When we are in a highly emotional state we tend to 'accept' the suggestions and they form a belief/program/pattern in our subconscious.

4) Just from observing our parents behaviors growing up, neural pathways or blueprints of beliefs were formed in our subconscious.

5) Hypnosis and NLP works simultaneously with both the subconscious and conscious mind acting as a bridge or a doorway to our subconscious mind.

"Suggestions given in a hypnotic state, even once, can produce actions in human beings that are the same type of actions that would have resulted in long-term conditioning and practice."

- An Institute of Cognitive and Neuroscience research study

Daily Gratitude Process

KEEP IT OR THROW IT AWAY BUT DO IT EVERYDAY

Taught to me by my mentor Blair Singer originally created by Allen Walter, his mentor.

GET A JOURNAL (ANY NOTEBOOK WILL WORK) AND WRITE ALL YOUR ANSWERS

1. **MAKE A DAILY GOAL -** This does not need to be measurable; Laugh more, learn something, be more patient
2. **WHAT AM I WILLING TO GIVE TO OTHERS TODAY?** – patience, energy, support, love, assistance
3. **WRITE 10 THINGS I FEEL GRATEFUL FOR OR COULD FEEL GRATEFUL FOR**
4. **WHAT AM I GRATEFUL FOR THAT SOMEONE ELSE DOES FOR ME?** Someone's trust in me, guidance
5. **WHAT AM I HAPPY ABOUT RIGHT NOW?** I got some sleep, I am alive, I have a computer

If you are feeling down or upset, focusing on gratitude can change you how you feel very quickly. Answering these 5 questions on a daily basis can truly help you feel good fast and help you to stay positive.

Sometimes when we are really down, you might need to ask yourself, "What *could* I feel grateful for instead of what do I feel grateful for?"

Two key components:

1. Actually feel the appreciation.
2. Make answering these questions a daily practice.

Use the next 2 pages to get you started. Enjoy!

DATE _____ **HYPNOSIS SESSION #** _____

My Experiences and insights from the hypnosis:

_____
_____
_____
_____
_____
_____
_____
_____
_____
_____
_____
_____
_____
_____
_____
_____
_____
_____
_____
_____
_____
_____
_____

<u>After the hypnosis session I felt:</u>
_____
_____

Affirming Statements or Mottos I will now verbalize every day:
_____
_____

I promise myself I will:

* _____
* _____
* _____

"YOU ARE ENOUGH!"

- It's an acceptance by the mind that something is true or real, often supported by an emotional or spiritual sense of certainty. It's similar to an all-knowing faith.

- A confidence in the truth or existence of something not immediately susceptible to rigorous proof.

Many of our beliefs that propel our lives were created by other people, and are false and self-limiting. If you wonder why you act the way do, it's because the fundamental behaviors, beliefs, values and attitudes we observed in our parents became hard-wired as neural pathways in our subconscious mind.

Our beliefs and values are the results of the environment we lived in while growing up. We accepted or rejected the experiences we observed. We modeled what we liked or rebelled against it. These experiences formed neural networks in our mind that we call programs or patterns. These beliefs/programs/patterns of behavior rule our lives. Our beliefs and values control us, even when they are someone else's belief and even if they are not based in truth!

We have many positive beliefs that we want to continue to reinforce with our thoughts. We also have negative and limiting beliefs that we need to release and change.

> *Discovering your limiting and negative beliefs*
> *gives you the opportunity to change them.*

It's a fascinating and uplifting experience when you stop judging yourself and your thoughts. You can really tune into negative beliefs that are holding you back from being your best self in every area of your life. Observe your thoughts and your beliefs. Recognize self-limiting beliefs and transform them to the truth. Remind yourself that you are made of the same innate intelligence that designed the Universe. You are an amazing creature whether you know it yet or not. It's time for you to acknowledge who you really are as well as the gifts you bring to those around you.

You Are Worthy!

As you do the exercise below, write the first words that pop into your head. (You might want to do this next part with a partner and have him/her read the word to you.) Just allow it to spark an immediate response. Have them write down your answers next to each word. Don't judge; be curious!

Women _____

Men _____

People _____

Sex _____

Love _____

Money _____

Work _____

Success _____

Failure _____

God _____

My Body _____

Weight Loss _____

Exercise _____

Smoking _____

Drinking _____

"What the mind can conceive and believe it can achieve."
- Napoleon Hill

Transform Limiting Beliefs into Empowering Beliefs

Write down your former limiting belief, cross it out and then write down your new empowering belief and all the benefits you will now experience as you honor your true self. Write it with a wonderful intention. Feel how it feels to be free. Say it in your mind and know it in your heart. Say it and own it many times a day.

Example

> **Limiting Belief –** *The old B.S. was that I can't heal myself.*
> **Empowering belief -** *The Truth is that I can heal myself. I am capable of healing myself.*
> **The Benefits -** *It's my destiny. I will have unlimited energy and clarity in helping others heal themselves completely. I will be able to create healing programs and tap into the healing energy.*

Limiting Belief _____

_____

<<< Empowering Belief >>><<< Empowering Belief >>>

The Benefits _____

_____

_____

_____

Limiting Belief _____

_____

<<< Empowering Belief >>><<< Empowering Belief >>>

The Benefits _____

_____

_____

_____

LIMITING BELIEF _____
_____

<<< EMPOWERING BELIEF >>><<< EMPOWERING BELIEF >>>

THE BENEFITS _____
_____
_____

LIMITING BELIEF _____
_____

<<< EMPOWERING BELIEF >>><<< EMPOWERING BELIEF >>>

THE BENEFITS _____
_____
_____
_____

LIMITING BELIEF _____
_____

<<< EMPOWERING BELIEF >>><<< EMPOWERING BELIEF >>>

THE BENEFITS _____
_____
_____
_____

DATE _____ **HYPNOSIS SESSION #** _____

My Experiences and insights from the hypnosis:

_____
_____
_____
_____
_____
_____
_____
_____
_____
_____
_____
_____
_____
_____
_____
_____
_____
_____
_____
_____
_____
_____
_____
_____

<u>After the hypnosis session I felt:</u>

_____
_____
_____

Affirming Statements or Mottos I will now verbalize every day:

_____
_____

I promise myself I will:

* _____
* _____
* _____

Self-Hypnosis

Research demonstrates that a daily hypnosis practice can improve your immune system, help you heal faster, gain more confidence and just create general feelings of personal well-being.

1. GET FOCUSED

What's your intention? What results will you picture in your mind? In other words, choose what you will focus on for the session.

The end result; the desired outcomes I want to experience in self-hypnosis are:

_____
_____
_____

2. BREATHE 3 TO 5 DEEP BELLY BREATHS
3. USE YOUR THOUGHTS AND INTENTIONS TO GUIDE YOURSELF INTO HYPNOSIS.
4. IMAGINE A SET OF 10 STAIRS — (OR USE YOUR FAVORITE INDUCTION)

Pretend you are the hypnotist and deliver suggestions to yourself going into hypnosis. Some examples of things you might say to yourself are:
- ❖ "Each step I go down, doubles my relaxation."
- ❖ "By the time I reach the bottom of the stairs I will feel 10 times more relaxed and become 10 times more focused."
- ❖ "I double my relaxation with every step I go down" or "I go deeper and deeper with every number."
- ❖ Tell yourself and feel yourself, "Relax, let go and go deeper, and deeper with every number, every step, or every level."

Use words between each number to guide yourself into a focused state. You can use the same words or change them. Give yourself suggestions to direct your mind and body.

5. CREATE YOUR PERSONALIZED 'MIND MOVIE'

Utilizing all your senses, vividly imagine yourself having the desired outcome; the end result with an incredibly wonderful feeling. Experience the desired outcome as it is already true.

During your mind movie **ENGAGE ALL YOUR SENSES.** Immerse yourself in the experience.

- ❖ Picture what you are wearing and exactly what you are doing. Imagine what other people are doing and saying. Be aware if you are inside or outside. Feel the ground beneath your feet. See the lights or the sun, plants/animals, etc.
- ❖ Hear everything that's going on, including what you are thinking and saying to yourself. Listen to what other people are saying to you. Hear the sounds of your environment; water, animals, music, etc.
- ❖ You may be able to smell and/or taste during the experience. Use these senses, too.
- ❖ The most IMPORTANT SENSE IS TO FEEL. FEEL the emotion, the passion, the gratitude, the inspiration, the confidence, the success, the happiness. **FEEL HOW GOOD IT FEELS** TO HAVE WHAT YOU WANT or be where you want to be. **FEEL** how good it feels to be 20 pounds lighter or **FEEL** how good it feels to have handled the situation well. **FEEL** how good it feels to be healthy. Use affirmations to confirm your feelings.

6. TAKE YOURSELF OUT OF HYPNOSIS

Count from 1 up to 5 and tell yourself that when you get to 5 you will open your eyes and feel wide-awake and great. And then begin counting. You can include words between each number that reinforce what you have done. 1, feeling confident 2, speeding up now calm, confident and in control 3, feeling great in every way 4, almost there and 5 open your eyes.

Forgiveness

"Forgiveness is a process that begins with learning and ends with loving yourself."
- Randi Light

Forgiveness is something you do for yourself. Forgiving frees you of negativity, doubt, worry, guilt and anger. It is not about condoning another person's behavior; it's about freeing you, so that you can be the best you can be. Hypnosis and NLP make it easier for you to clear the emotional charge, to neutralize the events and heal the wounds of the past so that you can create a bright and compelling future filled with love, peace and authenticity.

"If you are holding a grudge, a grudge is holding you."
– Inyanla Vanzant

When you love and accept yourself it's much easier to forgive yourself and forgive others. Forgiveness is a decision and a process in which you recognize your worthiness, regardless of what any human being ever did or said to you. As you begin to realize who you really are, you begin to accept the truth that 'YOU ARE WORTHY!' If you want to heal, you must let go of resentment, anger and guilt. Forgiveness is a process of awareness, learning, self love and acceptance.

"Forgiveness is for you, it's a gift to yourself. When you forgive, you set yourself free."
- Louise Hay

Once you recognize that you are holding on to negative feelings, you must learn to love yourself and believe in who you really are in order to let those feelings go. The reason you do it, is for you; so you can feel happy and fulfilled; so you can step into your power; so you can heal the wounds and in the process, heal your body, mind and spirit. Choose Forgiveness. You deserve to be free and happy. If you are ready, begin with the exercise below, if you are not sure, then read anything and everything you can about the effects of resentment, anger, guilt and forgiveness.

What do you believe forgiveness is?_____
_____
_____

What do you believe forgiveness does?_____
_____

How will not forgiving yourself or someone else affect your life?_____
_____
_____

What will forgiving yourself or someone else do for you?_____
_____
_____

Write down the names of some of the people that if you forgave, your life could look and feel better_____
_____

Do you love yourself enough to forgive and heal the wounds of your past?_____

Are you willing to forgive?_____
_____

"Until you heal the wounds of your past, you will continue to bleed into the future."
– Inyanla Vanzant

WHAT ARE YOU GOING TO DO TODAY TO FREE YOURSELF FROM THIS MENTAL AND PHYSICAL BURDEN THAT RESENTMENT AND GUILT HAS CREATED IN YOUR LIFE?

+ _____
+ _____
+ _____
+ _____

Learn + Love = Forgiveness

The purpose of this special report is to give your more clarity on the Art and Science of Forgiving so that you can live a happier and healthier life. Happiness is your birthright – don't allow anyone and their inappropriate behaviors take that away from you. Learn to Forgive and your birthright will begin to shine.

LEARN:

In order for you to truly feel happy and be your best self, you must forgive everyone and everything, including yourself. A key, strategic component of forgiveness is to learn from each and every life experience. When we can view the world, and each thing that takes place in our world, as a learning experience, it's easier to let go, move on and grow. When we learn, we feel better, change our 'state' and become resourceful. We can get through or over the situation faster and easier. I repeatedly ask myself, **"WHAT CAN I LEARN FROM THIS?"**

Something interesting to note is the way animals experience the world. Through their eyes, there is only the present, not the past, not the future- just the present. As a result, animals don't beat themselves up for past mistakes that happened last week or last year. They actually learn and move on. **YOU HAVE THAT ABILITY TOO!** We all have the ability to live more in the present and learn from each and every, and I mean each and every experience, from the little one's to the big ones.

"Self-Love means caring for ourselves enough, to forgive people in our past, so the wounds can no longer damage us-for the wounds do not hurt other people who hurt us, they hurt only us."
-Carolyn Myss

LOVE YOURSELF:

When we truly love ourselves, we stop judging ourselves harshly or judging ourselves by what other people did to us in the past. When you love yourself you can let go of the past and move forward. If our self worth is intact then we won't allow past or present perpetrators to affect our self-confidence. You might feel shaken up and unconfident for a brief period, but you don't stay in that state when you believe you are good enough. Unfortunately, very few people escaped childhood with the belief that they are good enough. If that's your case too, then it's time for you to use your thoughts, tools and resources to change your limiting beliefs to the truth. **YOU ARE GOOD ENOUGH!!!!!!!!!!!!** Repeat this statement every day, many times a day, **"I AM GOOD ENOUGH."** (Emphasize a different word each time.)

"Forgiveness is the answer to almost every problem."
- Louise Hay

FORGIVENESS:

At this point in your life, you may actually realize that forgiveness is for you, so you can live your life without the burdens and pains of resentment and guilt. When you forgive, it's for you, your healing and your happiness. I am talking about neutralizing your emotions, not condoning someone's behavior. You have an opportunity right now to heal, resolve and free yourself from your past wounds and hurts. Do you want to hold those grudges, no matter what the cost is to your health and your happiness? Or do you want to be happy and free to live your best life?

Some people seem to be able to naturally forgive while others just want to hold onto their history and how it affected them. The feeling that you are a victim holds you back and can literally ruin your life. Somehow, we create this false belief that we are hurting the perpetrator when we stay the victim. Nothing could be further from the truth!! Tony Robbins hit it right on the button when he said,

"Resenting another human being is like drinking poison and expecting your enemy to die."
- Tony Robbins

When a person acts inappropriate, it's usually because they have issues and need help, too. Even though we think it's about us, it's really not about us. If from your perspective and 'judgment' someone hurt *you* then you will continuously feel that pain like an open wound. The event could have been last week or 30 years ago, it doesn't matter, this wound still affects you and controls your beliefs and your actions. It helps to evaluate the experience and your role in it. It's also very important for you to learn to not take their 'stuff' personally and realize they have issues, too

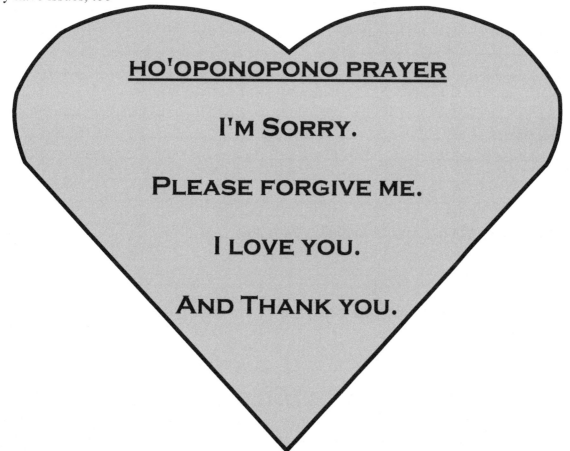

HO'OPONOPONO PRAYER

I'M SORRY.

PLEASE FORGIVE ME.

I LOVE YOU.

AND THANK YOU.

DATE _____ **HYPNOSIS SESSION #** _____

My Experiences and insights from the hypnosis:

_____
_____
_____
_____
_____
_____
_____
_____
_____
_____
_____
_____
_____
_____
_____
_____
_____
_____
_____
_____
_____
_____
_____
_____

<u>After the hypnosis session I felt:</u>

_____
_____
_____

Affirming Statements or Mottos I will now verbalize every day:

_____
_____

I promise myself I will:

* _____
* _____
* _____

Design Your Life!

WHAT WOULD YOU NEED TO HAVE DONE? WHO WOULD YOU NEEDED TO HAVE BECOME IN ORDER TO BE A PERSON YOU ARE DELIGHTED TO MEET ONE YEAR FROM TODAY?

Picture yourself walking along a beautiful and relaxing beach. You are enjoying the warmth of the sun and you see someone coming towards you walking confidently with grace and peace. All of the sudden you realize it's you, your future self, coming towards you. You admire your beauty, your clothes, and your body. You feel connected to your future self.

DESCRIBE WHO YOU MEET ON *(insert today's date)* _____

Include all the things you have accomplished and created emotionally, physically, mentally, spiritually and financially.

_____
_____
_____
_____
_____
_____
_____
_____
_____
_____
_____
_____
_____
_____
_____
_____
_____
_____
_____
_____
_____
_____
_____
_____
_____
_____
_____
_____
_____

GET FOCUSED

After meeting your future self, list what results or outcomes are most important to accomplish.
- ❖ _____
- ❖ _____
- ❖ _____
- ❖ _____
- ❖ _____

Why are these results important? What benefits will you get from achieving them?
- ❖ _____
- ❖ _____
- ❖ _____
- ❖ _____
- ❖ _____

IDEAS TO FACILITATE ACHIEVING YOUR GOALS

1. COMPLETE THE SMART GOALS BELOW.

2. HAND-WRITE (NOT ON YOUR COMPUTER) YOUR GOALS AS AFFIRMATIONS IN A JOURNAL EVERY DAY.

3. BEGIN ONE OF THE TASKS FOR EACH OF YOUR TOP 3 GOALS.

4. BEFORE YOU GO TO SLEEP AND WHEN YOU WAKE UP:

    A. GET INTO THAT ATTITUDE OF GRATITUDE

    B. PRACTICE THE SELF-HYPNOSIS TECHNIQUES

    C. VISUALIZE AND MATERIALIZE YOUR GOALS!

    D. SPEND APPROXIMATELY 30 MINUTES A DAY IN SELF-HYPNOSIS VISUALIZING YOURSELF ALREADY EXPERIENCING YOUR GOALS.

Do you know how to get what you want in life? Do you want to live with more passion and joy? Do you want more time, more energy, or more money? We live in a fast paced world. Sometimes we know what we want, but we can't seem to get it. Other times we are so confused by life's choices, we don't know what we want to do with our lives.

Flight Attendants remind us to put our oxygen masks on first and then help others. If you want to achieve greater amounts of joy and prosperity, you need to take care of and honor yourself. First, when we realize that nurturing ourselves is not a luxury, it's a necessity, we can think more clearly, have more energy and reduce many stressors.

"95% of people, who write down their goals and refer to them daily, accomplish them."
— Harvard Business School Study

S-M-A-R-T Goals

Specific, Measurable, Attainable, Realistic and Timely

When you know what you want and why you want it, it's much easier to get results. Now your mind has a target. The Law of Attraction is in action, only this time you are in the driver's seat.

A goal is a target. A goal is an outcome or a result you want to achieve or attain. You can focus on all areas of your life or just one specific area. Choose how you are going to proceed. Is this for your personal or professional life? I have listed categories you may want to include in your life plan.

Family, Job, Career, Health, Spiritual, Finances, Relationships, Healing, Emotional, Self

Example

Goal - "I want to stay calm in my interactions with my teenage son."

Why do you want this goal? Describe all the benefits that you will obtain from manifesting this outcome.

I will feel better. I will think clearer. Our relationship will be better. I will be a better role model. I will be a great example of how to respond in situations. My son will feel better about himself. My son will learn coping tools and techniques from my example. I will be less stressed.

What tasks will you begin doing to obtain this goal?

+ I will purchase Positive Discipline for Teenagers from *Amazon* on Wednesday morning.
+ On Thursday at 9:00am I will research information on communicating with teenagers.
+ I will take a deep breath and count to 3 before I respond in a conflict.
+ I will stop what I am doing, to communicate with him, so I am in better control of what I say consciously.

Turn your 'goal' into an affirmation so that it is in the present tense. Repeat it often; both out loud and to yourself.

"I am calm in my interactions with Noah."

Goal - _____

Why is this goal important? Describe all the benefits that you will obtain from manifesting this outcome.
_____
_____
_____

Describe the tasks you will begin doing now to obtain this goal.
_____
_____
_____
_____

Now, turn your goal into an affirmation so that it is in the present tense.
_____

Goal - _____

Why is this goal important? Describe all the benefits that you will obtain from manifesting this outcome.
_____
_____
_____

Describe the tasks you will begin doing now to obtain this goal.
_____
_____
_____
_____

Now, turn your goal into an affirmation so that it is in the present tense.
_____

Goal - _____

Why is this goal important? Describe all the benefits that you will obtain from manifesting this outcome.
_____
_____
_____

Describe the tasks you will begin doing now to obtain this goal.
_____
_____
_____
_____

Now, turn your goal into an affirmation so that it is in the present tense.
_____

Goal - _____

Why is this goal important? Describe all the benefits that you will obtain from manifesting this outcome.
_____
_____
_____

Describe the tasks you will begin doing now to obtain this goal.
_____
_____
_____
_____

Now, turn your goal into an affirmation so that it is in the present tense.
_____

DATE _____   **HYPNOSIS SESSION #** _____

My Experiences and insights from the hypnosis:

_____
_____
_____
_____
_____
_____
_____
_____
_____
_____
_____
_____
_____
_____
_____
_____
_____
_____
_____
_____
_____
_____
_____
_____

<u>After the hypnosis session I felt:</u> _____

_____
_____

Affirming Statements or Mottos I will now verbalize every day:

_____
_____

I promise myself I will:

* _____
* _____
* _____

DATE _____

Hypnosis – What it is and Why it's so effective

Hypnosis is a common everyday occurrence. Have you ever driven home and not remembered driving to your destination? Have you ever been so absorbed in a book or movie that you either felt the emotions of a character or forgot about your life for a period of time? These are examples of light states of hypnosis. *No one's clucking like a chicken!* You are just in a focused state.

Hypnosis is a focused state of awareness in which you naturally become more open to suggestion. Hypnosis is similar to meditation. Your brain waves slow down from the Beta state into Alpha and Theta. It's also a method of speaking to the innermost part of your mind, your subconscious, to eliminate old habits and behaviors and to generate new, beneficial behaviors. Research demonstrates that at least 95% of our behaviors are subconscious. In other words, our behaviors are a result of beliefs and emotions stored in our subconscious mind. We may not even be consciously aware of the beliefs and emotions behind our behaviors.

When your subconscious mind and conscious mind are in conflict, your subconscious mind overrides your conscious when it comes to making changes. Since hypnosis acts as a doorway, or a bridge, to the subconscious mind, we can access these patterns and limiting beliefs and ultimately change them. Hypnosis makes it easier and faster to release and let go of these subconscious belief systems.

When you are in a state of hypnosis you are more open to suggestion. In other words, positive suggestions are able to sink deeply into your subconscious mind more quickly and strongly than when you are in an "awake" state. Rest assured, only positive suggestions will work. All research has demonstrated that while in a hypnotic state, you cannot be made to do anything against your moral values. The Institute of Cognitive and Neuroscience has demonstrated that a suggestion given in a hypnotic state, even one time, can have the same effect as long-term conditioning and practice.

Hypnotists, also called hypnotherapists, do much more than provide positive suggestions. Many hypnotists have been trained in regression work. In other words, some hypnotists can regress you back in time to an experience that is the root cause or "source" of a physical problem or an emotional imprint. For instance, I was working with a client, who we shall call, Sarah. Sarah would grind her teeth at night. She wore a special brace to protect her teeth, yet the stress in her jaws muscles from trying to grind, lead to pain and headaches. To help relieve her, I guided her back in time to the root cause of her nighttime grinding. Sarah went back to an event in her life when she was a little girl and very scared. She was 7 years old, and in the kitchen where she grew up. Her father was angry and yelling. He actually broke the cabinet door and this scared her so much she ran to her bedroom to get away. Once at the source of the problem, I work with a variety of techniques including hypnotic reframing and inner child work, to help the little '7-year-old self' feel better and release the fear. That very night after the session, Sarah decided she wasn't going to wear her brace. When she awoke in the morning, she knew she hadn't been grinding her teeth because her jaw muscles had no tension and no pain. Regression is just one of many unique tools in the hypnotist's toolbox.

Hypnosis has been successfully used by millions of adults and children to improve athletic performance, sleep better, change limiting beliefs, stop worries, fears and other negative feelings, feel more confident in any situation, takeoff weight, stop smoking, improve memory, become more successful and so much more. Hypnosis has also been used as a complete anesthesia, in both childbirth and surgery. This means no chemicals and no side effects! For some people, just being able to reduce the amount of chemical anesthesia is extremely beneficial to their healing process.

The American Medical Association (AMA) and the American Dental Association approved hypnotherapy, also known as, the clinical use of hypnosis, in 1958. The American Psychological Association approved it shortly thereafter in 1960. It has been used in clinical settings for well over 150 years, around the world. In fact, the AMA believes hypnosis should be a part of every physicians training.

It is believed that we have over 60,000 thoughts per day! As we concentrate, our brain waves slow down. When we are present, or in the "now," we are more focused on what we are doing. These are examples of being in "The Zone," which is actually a light state of hypnosis. We are concentrating on hitting the golf ball, creating something unique or throwing the basketball into the net. When we enter "The Zone" we are definitely *not* talking to ourselves. Instead, we are intent on what we are doing which leads to much better results. Our brain waves are flowing in the Alpha state when we are in "The Zone." It's where all athletes do their very best.

NLP - Neuro-Linguistic Programming

"NLP is one of the biggest breakthroughs in the technology of achievement and human excellence."
-Time Magazine

NLP is a behavioral technology, which simply means that it is a set of guiding principles, attitudes and techniques. It allows you to change, adopt or eliminate fears, behaviors, allergies, and pains. NLP gives you the ability to choose your mental, emotional and physical states of well-being.

"NLP provides a systematic framework for directing our own brain. It teaches us how to direct not only our own states and behaviors, but also the states and behaviors of others. In short, it is the science of how to run your brain in an optimal way to produce the results your desire."
-Tony Robbins

"NLP is both an art and a scientific skill. Once the basic skills are mastered, it can be used for many things, for everything from medical hypnotherapy to excellence in sports, increasing study skills, relaxation for public speaking, and skill in business communications. It is a method of modeling excellence, a way of relaxing the body and increasing health, a set of therapy techniques modeled on the pioneering work of Milton Erickson, Fritz Perls, and Virginia Satir. It is a way of thinking and acting that easily generates rapport, easily changing the subconscious mind at deep levels, causing useful generative change. It quickens healing of physical ailments, rapidly removes emotional distress, and promotes deep peace and wellbeing. It gives an uncommon mastery of language patterns and a way to communicate simultaneously with a person's conscious and subconscious minds. More than all of these things, it is a way of being in the world in an artful way, fully present in the body, fully aware of the inner and outer senses, fully in possession of all one's of one's faculties and abilities, relaxed and ready for whatever lies ahead." *(The National Federation of Neuro-Linguistic Psychology)*

With NLP, you learn how to grow from every single life experience, thus increasing your ability to create a better quality of life

"NLP may be the most powerful vehicle for change in existence... NLP cannot be dismissed as just another hustle. It's theoretical underpinnings represent an ambitious attempt to codify and synthesize the insights of linguistics, body language, and the study of communication systems." *(Psychology Today)*

In our work together, NLP has been weaved into your sessions to help ensure your results. Below are some of the techniques you may have experienced during your training.

- TIME LINE THERAPY
- PARTS THERAPY
- ANCHORING
- CIRCLE OF POWER
- SWISH PATTERN
- NLP SUCCESS MODEL
- TOWARDS AND AWAY - MOTIVATION STRATEGY
- THE GODIVA TECHNIQUE
- REFRAMING
- HEALING AUTOMATICALLY
- THE FAST PHOBIA CURE
- FUTURE PACING
- CHANGING SUB MODALITIES
- MATCHING AND MIRRORING

These are tools, techniques and strategies that you can utilize on a regular basis to give you the ability to get access to what you want to feel and be each and every day. Take charge of your thoughts, feelings and actions. NLP can help you personally and professionally to live the life you really deserve.

Hypnosis Research

<u>Effectiveness of hypnosis as an adjunct to behavioral weight management.</u>**Journal of Clinical Psychology**, 41 (1), 35-41 - 109 17-67 year olds completed a behavioral treatment for weight management either with or without the addition of hypnosis. Results show that, at the end of the 9-week program, both interventions resulted in significant weight reduction. However, at 8-month and 2-year follow-ups, the hypnosis subjects showed significant additional weight loss, while those in the behavioral-treatment-only group exhibited little further change. More subjects who used hypnosis also achieved and maintained their personal weight goals. Bolocofsky, David N.; Spinler, Dwayne; Coulthard-Morris, Linda (1985).

<u>Hypnotherapy in weight loss treatment</u> **Journal of Consulting and Clinical Psychology.** Volume: 54 489-492 Investigated the effects of hypnosis in weight loss for 60 females, at least 20% overweight and not involved in other treatment....hypnosis was more effective than a control group (17 vs. .5 pounds on follow-up). Cochrane, Gordon; Friesen, J., (1986)

<u>Hypnotic enhancement of cognitive-behavioral weight loss treatments</u>**Journal of Consulting and Clinical Psychology,** 64 (3), 517-519.Averaged across post treatment and follow-up assessment periods, the mean weight loss was 6.00 lbs. (2.72 kg) without hypnosis and 11.83 lbs. (5.37 kg) with hypnosis....At the last assessment period, the mean weight loss was 6.03 lbs. (2.74 kg) without hypnosis and 14.88 lbs. (6.75 kg) with hypnosis... Correlational analyses indicated that the benefits of hypnosis increased substantially over time. Kirsch, Irving (1996).

Newer research from the University of Wisconsin shows <u>a meditation habit can strengthen the body's immune function, plus increase brain performance</u> in the form of electrical activity. It validates the mind-body dynamic of meditation. To gauge immune function, researchers measured antibodies in the blood that fight flu and other infections. Volunteer subjects who meditated had significantly higher levels of these healthful antibodies than non-meditators. By Bob Condor Tribune Newspapers

......"Hypnosis is real, says psychiatrist David Spiegel, a professor in the Department of Psychiatry and Behavioral Sciences at the Stanford University School of Medicine. It's no less palpable an analgesic than medication. Studies have confirmed these and other effects. Marie-Elisabeth Faymonville, an anesthetist at Leige University Hospital in Belgium, has used hypnosis during dozens of thyroidectomies, surgical removal of the thyroid gland. All her patients not only reported a very pleasant experience but had significantly less post-operative pain. They were also able to leave the hospital sooner and return to work faster than patients who received standard sedation for the same surgery, resulting in cost savings for hospitals and health-care insurers."

"HYPNOSIS WORKS" by Michael Abrams, Discover Magazine Winter 2008, The Brain page 64.

Excerpts: "The power of trance can no longer be disputed, a psychiatrist at Stanford says, it can ease pain, alter perception and sooth anxiety. Hypnotized subjects could resist intense pain for a full minute longer than those who weren't hypnotized. When highly hypnotizable subjects were asked to visualize colors, their brains responded just as if they actually were looking at them.

Sept. 25 (HealthDay News) <u>Hypnosis Cuts Hot Flashes for Breast Cancer Survivors</u> - Patients using the technique saw episodes diminish by 68%, study finds   -- Breast cancer survivors who suffer from hot flashes can reduce these attacks significantly with hypnosis, a new study finds. Women who underwent hypnosis had an average 68 percent decrease in the frequency and severity of hot flashes, the researchers found. In addition, these women said they experienced less anxiety and depression. They also had significant improvements in sleep and their ability to perform daily activities, compared with women who received no treatment.

"Hypnotic Hugs" by Hilary Waldman excerpt from an article in Hypnosis Today Magazine "Several large studies suggest that self-hypnosis helps children control bedwetting, procedure-related pain, headaches, and even asthma. One researcher in Ohio found that children with sickle cell disease used far fewer painkillers when they learned hypnosis to control their disease-related flare-ups.

The Questions We Ask

The questions we ask ourselves determine what we focus on and how we feel.

Step 1: Become aware of the questions you ask yourself.

Step 2: Change your questions to resourceful and useful ones.

Controlling how you feel at any given moment is key to your success and happiness. While we would love to never get into a negative state, the goal is to learn how to get in and out of that state quickly. Getting into an 'Attitude of Gratitude' is one way of changing how you feel for the better. Here are a few key ways you can change how you feel in any given moment.

- **Observing your thoughts instead of judging them.**
- **Tuning into the types of questions you are asking yourself.**
- **Asking resourceful and useful questions that will guide you to a more resourceful state.**

The following questions usually bring up uncomfortable feelings, yet many people play and replay these types of questions throughout the day.

> "Am I doing this right?"
>
> "Why does this always happen to me?"
>
> "Why am I so overweight?"
>
> "What's wrong with me?"

When you catch yourself asking these types of questions,
STOP ASKING THAT QUESTION AND CHANGE IT TO A MORE RESOURCEFUL QUESTION.

Becoming aware of the questions you ask yourself is an essential component to feeling happy, successful, and in control. Becoming aware of the questions we ask ourselves is an essential component in achieving lasting happiness.

The types of questions you ask determines the types of answers you get. When you ask yourself a resourceful question, you are naturally lead to resourceful answers. To change your focus, how you feel and the answers you think about in your mind, you must learn to ask yourself resourceful, results-oriented questions. By asking questions like this you actually feel better and create choices that lead you to discover many of the things you currently accept as unchangeable or out of your control, actually are changeable. Ask yourself outcome-based questions.

> **WHAT DO I NEED TO BELIEVE IN ORDER TO FEEL THIS WAY?**
>
> **WHAT CAN I DO ABOUT THIS SITUATION?**
>
> **WHAT CAN I LEARN FROM THIS?**
>
> **HOW CAN I MAKE THIS BETTER?**
>
> **WHAT DO I WANT? WHAT DO I REALLY WANT?**
>
> **WHAT RESOURCES DO I HAVE TO BEGIN MAKING CHANGES?**
>
> **WHAT CAN I DO RIGHT NOW TO FEEL BETTER?**
>
> **CAN I SEE ANY HUMOR IN THIS?**

Other resourceful questions that also help me gain control by changing my focus and my feelings:

- ❖ _____
- ❖ _____
- ❖ _____
- ❖ _____
- ❖ _____
- ❖ _____
- ❖ _____
- ❖ _____
- ❖ _____
- ❖ _____
- ❖ _____
- ❖ _____
- ❖ _____
- ❖ _____
- ❖ _____

Extra Worksheets

CHOOSE THE 6 MOST IMPORTANT ACTION STEPS FROM ALL 3 CATEGORIES THAT YOU COMMIT TO DO FOR TWO WEEKS. WRITE THEM AS AFFIRMATIONS.

Example: "I always picture myself at my new goal weight of 220."

1. _____

   _____

2. _____

   _____

3. _____

   _____

4. _____

   _____

5. _____

   _____

6. _____

   _____

Action Step #1 (write as an affirmation)

_____

_____

Today's date _____

Use the form below to track the days you complete your action step listed above. *Track your progress with check marks, smiley faces or any other way that makes you feel proud of yourself!*

SUN	MON	TUES	WED	THURS	FRI	SAT

Action Step #2 (write as an affirmation)

_____

_____

Today's date _____

Use the form below to track the days you complete your action step listed above. *Track your progress with check marks, smiley faces or any other way that makes you feel proud of yourself!*

SUN	MON	TUES	WED	THURS	FRI	SAT

Action Step #3 (write as an affirmation)

_____

_____

Today's date _____

Use the form below to track the days you complete your action step listed above. *Track your progress with check marks, smiley faces or any other way that makes you feel proud of yourself!*

SUN	MON	TUES	WED	THURS	FRI	SAT

Action Step #4 (write as an affirmation)

_____

_____

Today's date _____

Use the form below to track the days you complete your action step listed above. *Track your progress with check marks, smiley faces or any other way that makes you feel proud of yourself!*

SUN	MON	TUES	WED	THURS	FRI	SAT

Action Step #5 (write as an affirmation)

_____

_____

Today's date _____

Use the form below to track the days you complete your action step listed above. *Track your progress with check marks, smiley faces or any other way that makes you feel proud of yourself!*

SUN	MON	TUES	WED	THURS	FRI	SAT

Action Step #6 (write as an affirmation)

_____

_____

Today's date _____

Use the form below to track the days you complete your action step listed above. *Track your progress with check marks, smiley faces or any other way that makes you feel proud of yourself!*

SUN	MON	TUES	WED	THURS	FRI	SAT

Daily Accountability Ritual

Mental Training Reminder:
Our thoughts become our reality. What we think about most is what we manifest or bring into our lives. What you are focusing on naturally becomes a target therefore always focus on:

WHAT YOU WANT, WHAT YOU LIKE, WHAT YOU CAN DO AND WHAT YOU ARE GRATEFUL FOR.

BIG PICTURE GOAL _____

DAILY INTENTION _____

VIVIDLY IMAGINE THE INTENTION AND GOAL ALREADY COMPLETED WITH A GREAT FEELING FOR 1 MINUTE.

WHY I WANT THIS GOAL AND INTENTION.
_____
_____
_____
_____

CHECK IN WITH YOURSELF

1. I am feeling _____

2. Things I learned _____
_____
_____
_____

3. Little and big 'Wins' and accomplishments _____
_____
_____

4. Things I am doing and saying to take off weight and feel great _____
_____
_____

5. Things I no longer do or say to take off weight and feel great _____
_____
_____

6. Any self-sabotage or doubt that has gotten in my way _____
_____

7. Things I now do and say to override the little sabotaging voice _____
_____
_____

ENLIGHTENED LIVING HYPNOSIS, INC SERVICE AGREEMENT

1. Overview of Services. I am committed to helping you create your goals, achieve your goals, and heal in every way. Hypnosis and NLP (Neuro-Linguistic Programming) are some of the best tools for helping people make changes in their life. But just like anything else if life, you play a very important role in your own personal growth and healing. If I gave you a 'state of the art' shovel that was aerodynamic, great grip, light weight. and the perfect color; you may feel very grateful or you could believe there are better ones out there. In order for you to know how effective the tool is, you would need to use it regularly, get to know and understand it. By signing this agreement, I know that you are willing and ready to make the necessary changes and to practice the tools you learn during our sessions together.

2. Individual Level of Commitment.

Please circle your level of commitment in making changes in yourself and your life.

```
    0    1    2    3    4    5    6    7    8    9    10
Not ready                                          Very ready
```

3. Confidentiality. At Enlightened Living Hypnosis, I am committed to your success, therefore you can rest assured that this is a professional office and thereby holds strict standards of confidentiality.

4. Financial Policy. Full payment is due at the time of the service unless otherwise arranged. I offer a variety of programs and packages to ensure your success and to reduce the price per session. In order to provide a more economic package, I ask that you provide payment in full for the entire package. By cutting down on time dealing with payments, I can offer better rates. Be honest about your finances and if necessary we will set up a payment plan that is right for you.

5. Appointment Policy. **Any Session canceled without 24 hours notice is subject to a charge of $45**, less that half of the total for services rendered for one hypnosis session. "No Shows" will be charged the full price of the session. When rescheduling an appointment be sure to let me know immediately by **CALLING** me directly. **Please avoid email to let me know of scheduling changes.** This ensures I receive your change in a timely manner.

6. Something To Consider. After each session, most people feel very relaxed and leave my office with a renewed and fresh outlook on life. On occasion a session may bring up older issues that we have not yet resolved. Even though it is a natural response and part of the healing process, recognize that it could potentially make you feel uncomfortable. Since waiting until our scheduled appointment can seem too far away, if this were to occur please feel free to call or email me.

7. Personal Pledge. I understand that in order to be successful; I agree to listen to the hypnosis reinforcement CD's daily, complete the workbook, bring it to my sessions, practice the tools and techniques as well as keep my scheduled appointments because they are for my own personal growth and healing. By signing my name below, I accept a new path towards creating a better life for myself; therefore

I promise to do the best I can to stop self-criticism, stop getting down on myself and become my own BFF, Best Friend Forever.

By signing here, I understand and agree to the above terms.

Schedule of Sessions and Payments

Date_____   # of Sessions_____   Total Package Price_____

I agree to pay break the payments into   1   2   3   4   sessions, thereby paying in full when completed.

Payment 1   Check/Cash/CC: _____   Date Paid _____   Balance Due:_____

Payment 2   Check/Cash/CC: _____   Date Paid _____   Balance Due:_____

Payment 3   Check/Cash/CC: _____   Date Paid _____   Balance Due:_____

Payment 4   Check/Cash/CC: _____   Date Paid _____   Balance Due:_____

Dispute Resolution. Enlightened Living Hypnosis is committed to reducing internal and external conflicts and it is our belief that daily practice of the tools and techniques you receive at Enlightened Living Hypnosis should reduce internal and external conflicts. However, if a dispute arises out of this contract, and if the dispute cannot be settled through negotiation, the parties agree first to try in good faith to settle the dispute by mediation before resorting to arbitration, litigation, or some other dispute resolution procedure. The parties agree to use the Northern Indiana Better Business Bureau for the mediation process. The fees for the mediation will be borne equally by the parties.

When you purchase a package and pay in full, it reduces the costs per session. However if for some reason you cannot complete the number of sessions you committed to, you will be charged $300.00 for the first session and $250.00 for each additional session and not a discounted amount, for each session we worked together. Furthermore, you will be charged a service fee that includes credit card fees incurred plus a service or reimbursement fee of $60. You will also be charged for the CD and workbook at an additional price of $50.

I agree to the terms contained in this agreement and understand that they are binding. I further agree to pay the total amount as written above and agreed upon during the consultation.

Signed this_____(day) of_____(month), 20_____

_____
Recipient of Services

_____

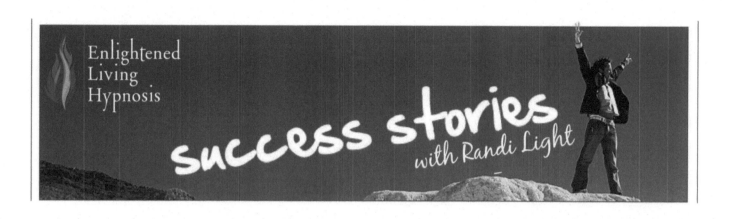

Success Stories with Randi Light

"Some of you know that I sent my daughter Sarah to see Randi Light for help with her Fibromyalgia, migraines, depression and sleep disorder. She is a different person! You might be skeptical but I can honestly tell you she is doing SO much better. She is waking up rested, happy, and practically pain free. She was skeptical going into it, but is a total believer now, as am I."

Mary Janiga

"Words cannot express how much you have helped change my life. I am sleeping better... I am much more positive everyday. The things from my past I am able to forgive in my heart — which I really never thought would happen. You are a true healer of life. I was skeptical in the beginning but let my heart guide me... I can make positive changes in my life — and have. Thank you. I went through 3 years of therapy and did not get the healing power like I did within 5 sessions with you."

~ Sara Sciarrabba
SendOutCards ~ www.WarmsYourHeart.com

"I did 3 sessions with Randi, one was over the phone at State. I was seated 8th place... We did some visualizations and I ended up shaving off 2 SECONDS from the 50 Meter Butterfly and getting 2nd at that meet. Later at Zones, I got the fastest time in the state for that season."

~ Jessica Yukich - Swimmer - Age 12

"Randi has helped change my way of thinking. She has worked with my children to help them overcome nightmares, and athletic competition challenges. I have personally used her services with excellent results. Several of those I care about have also utilized Randi's unique services and experienced extraordinary changes including overcoming fears, call reluctance, difficulty sleeping, weight loss, and more.

Not only does Randi help with all of the above, but she will teach you strategies for self help. I would highly recommend Randi and her services to anyone."

~ Carey Yukich, Wealth Manager - Airey Financial Group

"I was at a point in my life where I felt like I was going nowhere... From the very first meeting with you things started changing for the better. I am the happiest I've been in a long time. Through your hypnosis I have changed the way I approach everything in life and what it throws at me."

~ Matt Miller

"I came to see Randi for the first time 2 weeks ago. I was having a lot of trouble sleeping. I would wake up every night at 2:00 am and would be awake for 2 hours. Just from 1 session, I am sleeping through the night. If I wake up I turn over and fall right back asleep – That's amazing. I know longer let negativity into my life and I unconsciously choose not to let those things bother me. Because of that I found that I have a more positive attitude. And I am attacking the tasks of my workday with gusto. I have more business now than I have ever had before so I highly recommend that you invest in yourself and spend some time with Randi Light."

~ Susan Vukelich

© 2012 Randi Light • Enlightened Living Hypnosis, Inc. • All rights reserved